Depression

Everybody can feel miserable or overpowered now and again. However, misery is a constant sensation of void, bitterness, or failure to feel delight that might seem to occur for no great explanation. It is unmistakable from distress and different feelings an individual might feel following troublesome life altering situations.

By

Fredrick Eben

Copyright ©

Table of contents

Introduction

Despondency is the main source of handicap around the world.

It can subvert an individual's connections, make working and keeping up with great well being extremely challenging, and in serious cases, may prompt self destruction. As a matter of fact, sadness adds to almost 40,000 suicides in the United States every year.

It can influence grown-ups, young people, and kids. This article inspects what discourages and causes it, as well as sorts of sorrow, treatment, and that's only the tip of the iceberg.

Chapter one

What is depression?

Misery is a temperament problem that causes tenacious sensations of trouble, vacancy, and loss of happiness. Unique in relation to the temperament vacillations individuals routinely experience as a piece of life.

Significant life altering situations, like mourning or the passing of a task, can set off sorrow. Yet, sorrow is particular from the pessimistic sentiments an individual may briefly have in light of a troublesome life altering situation.

Misery frequently perseveres regardless of a difference in conditions and causes sentiments that are extreme, constant, and not relative to an individual's conditions.

It is a continuous issue, not a passing one. While there are various kinds of sorrow, the most well-known one is a significant and burdensome problem. It comprises episodes during which the side effects keep going for no less than about fourteen days.

Wretchedness can keep going for a little while, months, or years. For some individuals, a persistent disease improves and afterward backslides.

Is it repairable?
While there is no solution for sadness, there are viable medicines that assist with recuperation. The earlier that treatment begins, the more fruitful it could be. Certain individuals might in all likelihood at no point ever experience melancholy in the future after a solitary time of it. Others will keep on having backslides.

Many individuals encountering despondency recuperate after a treatment plan. Indeed, even with compelling treatment, in any case, a backslide may happen. About a portion of individuals don't at first answer treatment.

To forestall backslide, individuals who take prescription for sadness ought to go on with treatment — even after side effects improve or disappear — however long their primary care physician prompts.

Signs and side effects
Gloom can cause a scope of mental and actual side effects, including:

•persevering discouraged state of mind

•loss of interest or delight in leisure activities and exercises

•changes in craving and body weight

•strangely sluggish or unsettled developments

•diminished energy or weakness

•trouble resting or sleeping in

•unreasonable sensations of responsibility or uselessness

•trouble focusing or simply deciding

•considerations of death or self destruction, or self destruction endeavors.

On the off chance that an individual encounters at least five of these side effects during a similar 2-week time frame, a specialist might determine them to have misery.

Wretchedness may likewise cause different side effects, including peevishness, fretfulness, ongoing agony, migraines, and stomach related issues.

Kinds of wretchedness
There are a few types of wretchedness. The following are probably the most widely recognized types.

✓Significant gloom

An individual living with significant gloom encounters a consistent mindset of trouble. They might lose interest in exercises they used to appreciate.
Treatment typically includes prescription and psychotherapy.

✓Diligent burdensome issue

Otherwise called dysthymia, diligent burdensome issues cause side effects that keep going for something like 2 years.

An individual living with this issue might have episodes of significant gloom as well as milder side effects that don't meet the rules for significant burdensome problems.

✓Post pregnancy anxiety

In the wake of conceiving an offspring, certain individuals experience a short time of bitterness or elevated feelings that certain individuals call the "blue eyes." This generally disappears in a couple of days to half a month.

Postpartum anxiety, or postpartum anxiety, is more serious.

There is no single reason for this kind of melancholy, and it can endure for months or years. Any individual who encounters progressing sorrow after conveyance ought to look for clinical consideration.

Significant burdensome issue with occasional example

Recently known as occasional full of feeling problems (SAD), this sort of melancholy ordinarily happens throughout the colder time of year and fall months, when there is less sunshine. Less normally, it might follow other occasional examples.

It lifts during the remainder of the year and because of light treatment.

This condition appears to especially influence individuals who live in nations with long or extreme winters.

What causes discouragement?
The clinical local area doesn't completely figure out the reasons for despondency. There are numerous potential causes, and some of the time, different variables join to set off side effects.

Factors that are probably going to assume a part include:

•hereditary elements

•changes in the mind's synapse levels

•natural factors like openness to injury or absence of social help

•mental and social variables

•extra circumstances, like bipolar issue

Connections between different variables can expand the gamble of sadness. For example, an individual with a family ancestry or a hereditary gamble of misery might encounter side effects of despondency following a horrible mishap.

The side effects of misery can include:

•a discouraged state of mind
•decreased interest or joy in exercises that an individual recently delighted in
•a deficiency of sexual craving
•changes in craving
•inadvertent weight reduction or gain
•resting excessively or excessively little
•unsettling, fretfulness, and pacing all over
•eased back development and discourse
•exhaustion or loss of energy
•sensations of uselessness or culpability

•trouble thinking, focusing, or simply deciding

•intermittent considerations of death or self destruction, or an endeavor at self destruction

In females
Misery is almost two times as normal in females than guys, as per the Centers for Disease Control and Prevention (CDC).

Analysts don't have any idea why despondency gives off an impression of being more normal in females. Nonetheless, a recent report suggests that the distinction might be because of differences in detailing. Specialists observed that females were almost certain than guys to report and look for treatment for sorrow side effects.

Some examination proposes that openness to orientation separation builds the gamble of misery.

Additionally, a few kinds of despondency are novel to females, like post pregnancy anxiety and premenstrual dysphoric issues.

In guys
As per information from the National Health and Nutrition study, which depends on self-reports of psychological well-being side effects, 5.5% of guys report sadness side effects in a given 2-week time span, compared to 10.4% of females.

Guys with discouragement are more probable than females to savor liquor overabundance, show outrage, and participate in risk-taking because of the problem.

Different side effects of gloom in guys might include:

•keeping away from family and social circumstances
•working without a break

•experiencing issues staying aware of work and family obligations
•showing oppressive or controlling conduct in connections

In undergrads
Time at school can be upsetting, and an individual might be managing different ways of life, societies, and encounters interestingly.

A few understudies experience issues adapting to these changes, and they might foster sorrow, nervousness, or both subsequently.

Side effects of sadness in understudies might include:

•trouble focusing on homework
sleep deprivation
•resting excessively
•a reduction or expansion in hunger
•staying away from social circumstances and exercises that they used to appreciate

In teenagers
Actual changes, peer pressure, and different elements can add to gloom in teens.

They might encounter a portion of the accompanying side effects:

•feeling touchy
•fretfulness, for example, a failure to stand by
•pulling out from loved ones
•trouble focusing on homework
•feeling regretful, powerless, or useless

In youngsters
That's what the CDC gauge, in the U.S., 4.4% of youngsters and teens matured 3-17 have a finding of sorrow. This figure has risen lately.

Despondency in kids can make homework and social exercises testing. They might encounter side effects, for example,

•crying

•low energy

•tenacity

•insubordinate way of behaving

•vocal eruptions

More youthful kids might experience issues communicating how they feel in words. This can make it harder for them to make sense of their sensations of bitterness.

In generally underestimated gatherings
Research shows that the predominance of significant despondency among African Americans has been around 10.4%, contrasted and 17.9% among individuals who are white.

Be that as it may, 56% of African Americans experience despondency all the more constantly, contrasted and 38.6% of individuals who are white. This suggests that however less African Americans might encounter gloom, the people who really do may encounter it for longer. Moreover, not exactly 50% of these African Americans have looked for treatment.

Other examinations demonstrate that African Americans might have melancholy less of the time than non-Hispanic individuals who are white, yet this might be because of the way that numerous African Americans frequently don't have a legitimate conclusion.

Chapter two

Triggers

Triggers are close to home, mental, or actual occasions or conditions that can make gloomy side effects show up or return.

These are probably the most well-known triggers:

•upsetting life altering situations, for example, misfortune, family clashes, and changes in connections

•deficient recuperation in the wake of having halted despondency treatment too early

•ailments, particularly a clinical emergency, for example, another conclusion or a constant sickness like coronary illness or diabetes

Risk factors

Certain individuals have a higher gamble of discouragement than others.

Risk factors include:

•encountering specific life altering situations, for example, deprivation, work issues, changes in connections, monetary issues, and clinical worries

•encountering intense pressure

•having an absence of effective ways of dealing with especially difficult times

•having a direct relation with melancholy

•utilizing a few physician recommended drugs, like corticosteroids, certain beta-blockers, and interferon

•utilizing sporting medications, like liquor or amphetamines

•having supported a head injury

•having a neurodegenerative infection like Alzheimer's or alternately Parkinson's

•having had a past episode of significant misery

•having a constant condition, like diabetes, ongoing obstructive pneumonic illness (COPD), or cardiovascular sickness

•living with constant torment

•lacking social help

Sadness as a side effect
Sadness can likewise happen as a side effect or comorbidity with another emotional well-being condition. Models include:

Crazy despondency
Psychosis can include hallucinations, like deceptions and a separation from the real world. It can likewise include mind flights — detecting things that don't exist.

Certain individuals experience melancholy with psychosis. An individual living with psychosis, which is a serious mental disease, may encounter sadness therefore.

On the other hand, an individual living with discouragement might have a serious type of the condition that likewise incorporates psychosis side effects.

Bipolar confusion
Discouragement is a typical side effect of bipolar problems. Individuals with bipolar confusion experience times of melancholy that might last weeks. They likewise experience times of craziness, which is a raised state of mind that might make an individual vibe exceptionally blissful, forceful, or crazy.

Treatment
Discouragement is treatable, however the treatment might rely upon the specific kind an individual is living with.

Be that as it may, around 30.9% of individuals don't answer treatment or answer ineffectively. Around 4 out of 10 individuals accomplish reduction of their side effects in no less than a year, yet melancholy can return.

Overseeing side effects as a rule includes three parts:

◆Support: This can go from examining down to earth arrangements and potential causes to teaching relatives.

◆Psychotherapy: Also known as talking treatment, a few choices incorporate balanced guiding and mental social treatment (CBT).

◆Drug treatment: A specialist might recommend antidepressants.

Drug

Antidepressants can assist with getting moderate extreme gloom. A few classes of antidepressants are accessible:

•particular serotonin reuptake inhibitors (SSRIs)

•particular serotonin and norepinephrine reuptake inhibitors (SNRIs)

•abnormal antidepressants

•tricyclic antidepressants

•monoamine oxidase inhibitors (MAOIs)

Each example of genuine greatness on an alternate synapse or blend of synapses.

An individual ought to just accept these drugs as their primary care physician recommends. A few medications can require a long time to have an effect. By halting taking the medication, an individual may not encounter the advantages that it can offer.

Certain individuals quit taking prescriptions after side effects improve, however this can prompt a backslide.

An individual ought to raise any worries about antidepressants with a specialist, including any goal to quit taking the prescription.

Drug incidental effects
SSRIs and SNRIs can make side impacts. An individual might insight:

•sickness
•blockage
•loose bowels
•low glucose
•weight reduction or weight gain
•a rash
•sexual brokenness

The Food and Drug Administration (FDA) expects producers to put a "black box" cautioning on upper containers.

That's what the admonition shows, among different dangers, these drugs might increment self-destructive contemplations or activities in certain kids, teens, and youthful grown-ups inside the initial not many long periods of treatment. While there is an expansion in risk, the outright gamble stays low.

Chapter three

Food and diet

Some exploration proposes that eating a great deal of sweet or handled food varieties can prompt different actual medical issues and poor emotional wellness. Consequences of a recent report recommend that an eating routine that incorporates a considerable lot of these kinds of food can influence the emotional well-being of youthful grown-ups.

The investigation additionally discovered that eating a greater amount of the accompanying food sources decreased wretchedness side effects:

•natural product
•vegetables
•fish
•olive oil

Psychotherapy

Psychotherapy, or talking treatments, for despondency incorporate CBT, relational psychotherapy, and critical thinking treatment.

For certain types of despondency, psychotherapy is typically the first-line treatment, while certain individuals answer better to a blend of psychotherapy and meds.

CBT and relational psychotherapy are the two primary kinds of psychotherapy for misery. An individual might have CBT in individual meetings with a specialist, in gatherings, via phone, or on the web.

CBT centers around assisting an individual with recognizing the association between their viewpoints, ways of behaving, and sentiments. They then work consistently to change hurtful considerations and ways of behaving.

Relational treatment means to assist individuals with recognizing:

•profound issues that influence connections and correspondence

•what these issues additionally mean for their temperament

•the most effective method to further develop connections and better deal with feelings

Work out

Vigorous activity raises endorphin levels and invigorates synapses, possibly facilitating melancholy and uneasiness. A 2019 paper expresses that exercise might be particularly useful with treatment-safe gloom.

Practice offers the best advantages when an individual consolidates it with standard medicines, like antidepressants and psychotherapy.

Cerebrum feeling treatments
Cerebrum feeling treatments are another treatment choice. For instance, dull

transcranial attractive feelings send attractive heartbeats to the mind, and this might assist with treating significant sadness.

In the event that downturn doesn't answer drug treatment, an individual might profit from electroconvulsive treatment (ECT). Specialists don't completely comprehend how ECT functions.

During the method, an individual is snoozing, and a specialist utilizes power to incite a seizure. This might help "reset" the cerebrum, rectifying issues with synapses or different issues that cause misery.

Conclusion
Assuming an individual suspects that they have side effects of sorrow, they ought to look for proficient assistance from a specialist or psychological wellness subject matter expert.

A certified wellbeing expert can preclude different causes, guarantee an exact conclusion, and give protected and successful treatment.

They will pose inquiries about side effects, for example, how long they have been available. A specialist may likewise direct an assessment to check for actual causes and request a blood test to preclude other medical issues.

Is despondency hereditary?
An individual with a parent or kin who has discouragement is multiple times more probable than others to foster the condition.

Be that as it may, many individuals with discouragement have no family background of it.

A new report proposes that vulnerability to sadness may not outcome from hereditary variety. The analysts recognize that while individuals can acquire sorrow, numerous different issues likewise impact its turn of events.

FAQ

What does sorrow do to the cerebrum?
Sadness can prompt changes in degrees of synapses, which are atoms that communicate messages between nerve cells. Over the long haul, it might likewise make actual changes to the cerebrum, remembering decreases for dim matter volume and expanded irritation.

Does melancholy change your character?
Research has turned up blended results about whether wretchedness can really change an individual's character.

In any case, as per one audit of 10 examinations, burdensome side effects might be related with changes in a few explicit parts of character — including extraversion, neuroticism, and suitability — which could be transitory or diligent.

Does melancholy influence your reasoning? Melancholy can modify focus and independent direction. It might likewise impede consideration and cause issues with data handling and memory.

Outline

Despondency is a serious, constant ailment that can influence each part of an individual's life. At the point when it causes self-destructive considerations, it tends to be deadly.

Individuals can't think right out of gloom. Melancholy is definitely not an individual coming up short or an indication of shortcoming. It is treatable, and looking for treatment early may build the possibilities of recuperation.

Since wretchedness can be trying to treat, an individual must see a specialist with skill in sorrow and to attempt a few distinct medicines. Frequently, a blend of treatment and drug offers the best outcomes.